Keto Diet for fit and healthy women

Lose Weight without sacrificing taste

Hollie Armstrong

TABLE OF CONTENTS

Readers acknowledge that the author is not engaging in the rendering of legal, financial, medical or professional advice. The content within this book has been derived from various sources. Please consult a licensed professional before attempting any techniques outlined in this book. By reading this document, the reader agrees that under no circumstances is the author responsible for any losses, 5 direct or indirect, which are incurred as a result of the use of information contained within this document, including, but not limited to, — errors, omissions, or inaccuracies.

BREAKFAST

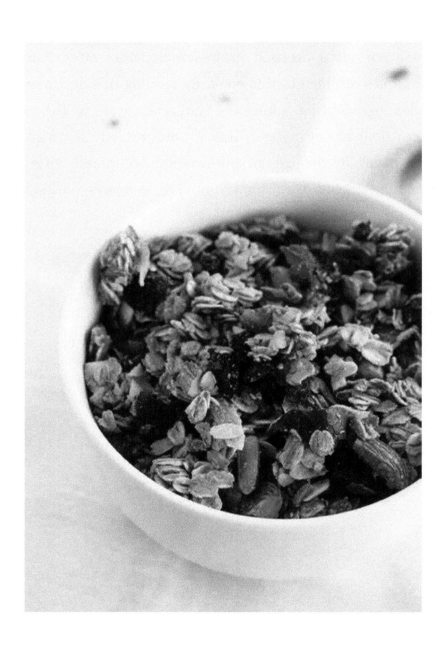

Simple Egg Porridge

Servings: 2

Cooking Time: 4 minutes

Ingredients

- 2 eggs
- 1 tablespoon stevia
- 1/3 cup heavy cream
- 2 tablespoons ghee, melted
- A pinch of cinnamon, ground

Directions:

1. In a bowl, mix eggs with stevia and heavy cream and whisk well.
2. Heat up a pan with ghee over medium-high heat, add egg mixture and cook until they are done.
3. Transfer to 2 bowls, sprinkle cinnamon on top and serve.
4. Enjoy!

Nutrition Info:

Calories 340, fat 12, fiber 10, carbs 3, protein 14

Amazing Chicken Omelet

Servings: 1

Cooking Time: 10 minutes

Ingredients

- 1-ounce rotisserie chicken, shredded
- 1 teaspoon mustard
- 1 tablespoon homemade mayonnaise
- 1 tomato, chopped
- 2 bacon slices, cooked and crumbled
- 2 eggs
- 1 small avocado, pitted, peeled and chopped
- Salt and black pepper to the taste

Directions:

1. In a bowl, mix eggs with some salt and pepper and whisk gently.
2. Heat up a pan over medium heat, spray with some cooking oil, add eggs and cook your omelet for 5 minutes.
3. Add chicken, avocado, tomato, bacon, mayo and mustard to one half of the omelet.
4. Fold omelet, cover the pan and cook for 5 minutes more.
5. Transfer to a plate and serve.
6. Enjoy!

Nutrition Info: calories 400, fat 32, fiber 6, carbs 4, protein 25

Incredible Breakfast Salad in a Jar

Servings: 1

Cooking Time: 0 minutes

Ingredients

- 1-ounce favorite greens
- 1-ounce red bell pepper, chopped
- 1-ounce cherry tomatoes halved
- 4 ounces rotisserie chicken, roughly chopped
- 4 tablespoons extra virgin olive oil
- ½ scallion, chopped
- 1-ounce cucumber, chopped
- Salt and black pepper to the taste

Directions:

1. In a bowl, mix greens with bell pepper, tomatoes, scallion, cucumber, salt, pepper and olive oil and toss to coat well.
2. Transfer this to a jar, top with chicken pieces and serve for breakfast.
3. Enjoy!

Nutrition Info: calories 180, fat 12, fiber 4, carbs 5, protein 17

Mint & Cocoa Smoothie
Servings: 2

Cooking Time: 5 minutes

Ingredients

- 1/3 ripe avocado, peeled and pitted
- 3 teaspoons cacao powder, unsweetened
- 1/4 teaspoon grated nutmeg
- 2 teaspoons granulated erythritol
- 1 cup milk
- 1/2 cup water

Directions:

1. Puree all ingredients in a blender until smooth and uniform.

2. Spoon into two glasses and enjoy!

Nutrition Info (Per Serving):

140 Calories; 9g Fat; 6.6g Carbs; 3.7g Protein; 2.8g Fiber

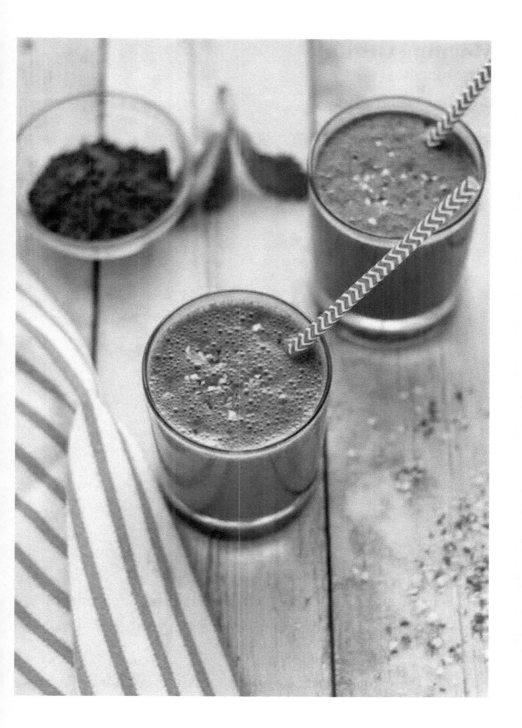

Morning Granola

Servings: 8

Cooking Time: 1 Hour

Ingredients

- 1 tbsp coconut oil
- ⅓ cup almond flakes
- ½ cup almond milk
- ½ tbsp liquid stevia
- 1/8 tsp salt
- 1 tsp lime zest
- 1/8 tsp nutmeg, grated
- ½ tsp ground cinnamon
- ½ cup pecans, chopped
- ½ cup almonds, slivered
- 2 tbsp pepitas
- 3 tbsp sunflower seeds
- ¼ cup flax seed

Directions:

1. Set a deep pan over medium heat and warm the coconut oil. Add almond flakes and toast for about 2 minutes. Stir in the remaining ingredients.

2. Set the oven to 300° F. Lay the mixture in an even layer onto a baking sheet lined with parchment paper. Bake for

1 hour, making sure that you shake gently in intervals of 15 minutes. Serve alongside additional almond milk.

Nutrition Info (Per Serving): Kcal 262; Fat: 24.3g, Net Carbs: 9.2g, Protein: 5.1g

BRUNCH

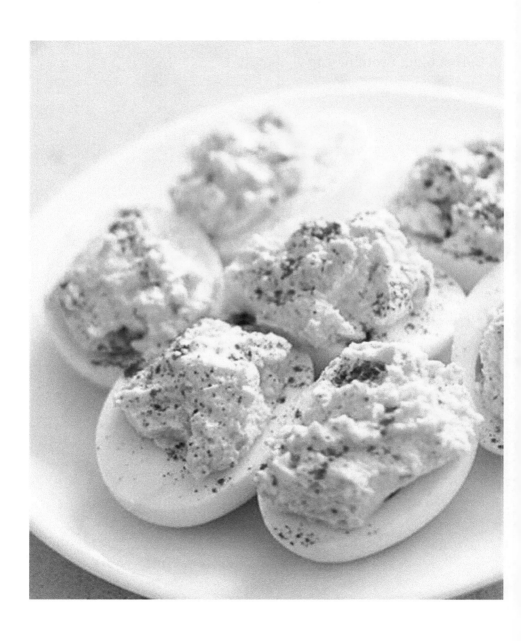

Yogurt Deviled Eggs

Servings: 2

Cooking Time: 0 minutes

Ingredients

- 2 eggs, boiled
- 1/8 tsp paprika
- 1 tsp mustard paste
- 1 tsp soy sauce
- 2 tbsp yogurt
- Seasoning:
- ¼ tsp salt
- 1/8 tsp ground black pepper

Directions:

1. Peel the boiled eggs, then slice in half lengthwise and transfer egg yolks to a medium bowl by using a spoon.
2. Mash the egg yolk, add remaining ingredients and mash until smooth and well combined.
3. Spoon the egg yolk mixture into egg whites, sprinkle with some more paprika and then serve.

Nutrition Info: 95 Calories; 6 g Fats; 7.6 g Protein; 1.2 g Net Carb; 0.1 g Fiber;

Baked Chorizo with Cottage Cheese

Servings: 6

Cooking Time: 30 minutes

Ingredients

- 7 oz Spanish chorizo, sliced
- 4 oz cottage cheese, pureed
- ¼ cup chopped parsley

Directions:

1. Preheat the oven to 325 F. Line a baking dish with waxed paper. Bake the chorizo for minutes until crispy.

2. Remove from the oven and let cool. Arrange on a Serves platter.

3. Top each slice with cottage cheese and parsley.

Nutrition Info (Per Serving): Cal 172; Net Carbs: 0.2g; Fat: 13g; Protein: 5g

Mini Salmon Bites

Servings: 10

Cooking Time: 15 minutes

Ingredients

- 8 ounces cream cheese, softened
- 4 ounces smoked salmon, chopped
- 2 medium scallions, thinly sliced
- Bagel seasoning, as required

Directions:

1. In a bowl, add the cream cheese and beat until fluffy.
2. Add the smoked salmon and scallions and beat until well combined. Make bite-sized balls from the mixture and lightly coat with the bagel seasoning.
3. Arrange the balls onto 2 parchment-lined baking sheets and refrigerate for about 2-3 hours before serving.
4. Enjoy!

Nutrition Info (Per Serving): Calories: 94; Net Carbs: 0.7g; Carbohydrate: 0.8g; Fiber: 0.1g; Protein: 3.8g; Fat: 8.4g; Sugar: 0.1g; Sodium: 294mg

Easy Caprese Appetizer

Servings: 8

Cooking Time: 10 minutes

Ingredients

- 2 tablespoons extra-virgin olive oil
- 2 tablespoons red wine vinegar
- 1 tablespoon Italian seasoning blend
- 8 pieces Prosciutto
- 8 pieces Soppressata
- 16 grape tomatoes
- 8 black olives, pitted
- 8 ounces mozzarella, cubed
- 2 tablespoons fresh basil leaves, chopped
- 1 red bell pepper, sliced
- 1 yellow bell pepper, sliced
- Coarse sea salt, to taste

Directions:

1. In a small mixing bowl, make the vinaigrette by whisking the oil, vinegar, and Italian seasoning blend. Set aside.
2. Slide the ingredients on the prepared skewers.
3. Arrange the sticks on a serving platter. Season with salt to taste. Serve the vinaigrette on the side and enjoy!

Nutrition Info (Per Serving): 141 Calories; 8.2g Fat; 3.3g Carbs; 12.9g Protein; 1g Fiber

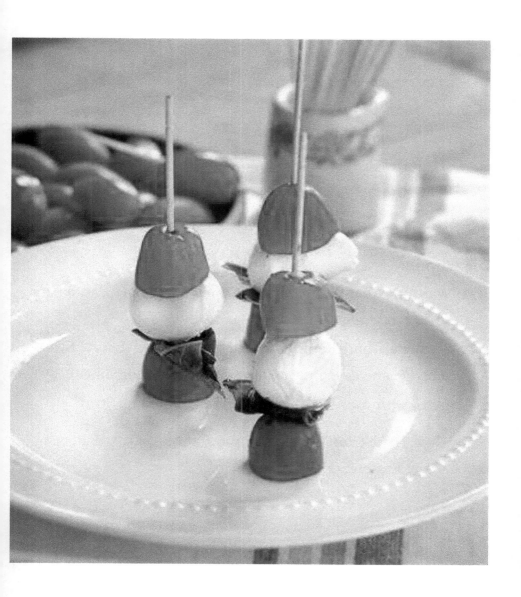

Swiss Cheese Dip

Servings: 8

Cooking Time: 10 minutes

Ingredients

- 1 cup double cream
- 4 ounces Ricotta cheese
- 4 tablespoons Greek yogurt
- 8 ounces Swiss cheese, shredded
- Cayenne pepper, to taste

Directions:

1. Warm the double cream and Ricotta cheese in a sauté pan over moderate heat.
2. Remove from the heat. Fold in the Greek yogurt, Swiss cheese, and cayenne pepper. Gently stir to combine.
3. Serve with your favorite keto dippers. Bon appétit!

Nutrition Info (Per Serving): 196 Calories; 15.7g Fat; 3.4g Carbs; 10.1g Protein; 0g Fiber

SOUP AND STEWS

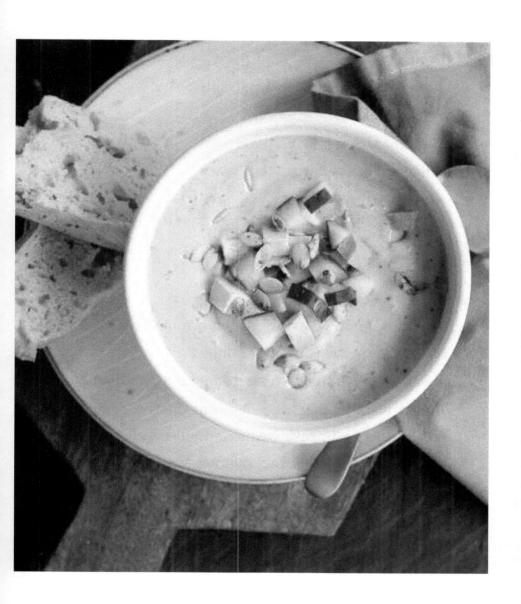

Delicious Avocado Soup

Servings: 4

Cooking Time: 10 minutes

Ingredients

- 2 avocados, pitted, peeled and chopped
- 3 cups chicken stock
- 2 scallions, chopped
- Salt and black pepper to the taste
- 2 tablespoons ghee
- 2/3 cup heavy cream

Directions:

1. Heat up a pot with the ghee over medium heat, add scallions, stir and cook for 2 minutes.
2. Add and ½ cups stock, stir and simmer for 3 minutes.
3. In your blender, mix avocados with the rest of the stock, salt, pepper and heavy cream and pulse well. Add this to the pot, stir well, cook for 2 minutes and season with more salt and pepper.
4. Stir well, ladle into soup bowls and serve.
5. Enjoy!

Nutrition Info: calories 332, fat 23, fiber 4, carbs 6, protein 6

Summer Tomato Soup

Servings: 4

Cooking Time: 40 minutes

Ingredients

- 2 cloves garlic, finely sliced
- 1/2 large red onion, finely chopped
- 2 tablespoons olive oil
- salt and pepper, to taste
- 1 ½ tablespoon tomato paste
- 2 cups tomatoes, peeled and diced
- 2 celery stalks, peeled and chopped
- 2 cups vegetable broth
- 1/3 teaspoon paprika
- 1/3 teaspoon oregano
- ½ cup heavy cream
- ½ teaspoon dried basil
- ½ cup parmesan cheese, shredded

Directions:

1. Heat the olive oil in a large pot, add the garlic, celery, and red onion. Cook for 2-3 minutes.
2. Then stir in the tomatoes, tomato paste, and vegetable broth. Season with salt, pepper, paprika, oregano, and basil. Boil for -25 minutes or until the tomatoes are soft.

3. Remove from the heat and blend with an immersion blender. Stir in the heavy cream and continue to boil for 1-2 minutes.

4. Serve in bowls and top with parmesan cheese.

Nutrition Info (Per Serving): 202 Calories; 16.1g Fat; 7g Carbs; 1.8g Fiber; 6g Protein

Creamy Asparagus Soup

Preparation Time: 10 minutes

Cooking Time: 15 minutes

Servings: 4

Ingredients:

- lbs. asparagus, cut the ends and chop into 1/2-inch pieces
- 2 tbsp. olive oil
- garlic cloves, minced
- 2 oz parmesan cheese, grated
- 1/2 cup heavy cream
- 1/4 cup onion, chopped
- 4 cups vegetable stock
- Pepper
- Salt

Directions:

1. Heat olive oil in a large pot over medium heat.
2. Add onion to the pot and sauté until onion is softened. Add asparagus and sauté for 2-3 minutes.
3. Add garlic and sauté for a minute. Season with pepper and salt.
4. Add stock and bring to boil. Turn heat to low and simmer until asparagus is tender.

5. Remove pot from heat and puree the soup using an immersion blender until creamy.

6. Return pot on heat. Add cream and stir well and cook over medium heat until just soup is hot. Do not boil the soup.

7. Remove from heat. Add cheese and stir well. Serve and enjoy.

Nutrition:

Calories: 202 Fat: 8.4g Fiber: 6.1g Carbohydrates: 3.1 g Protein: 5.3g

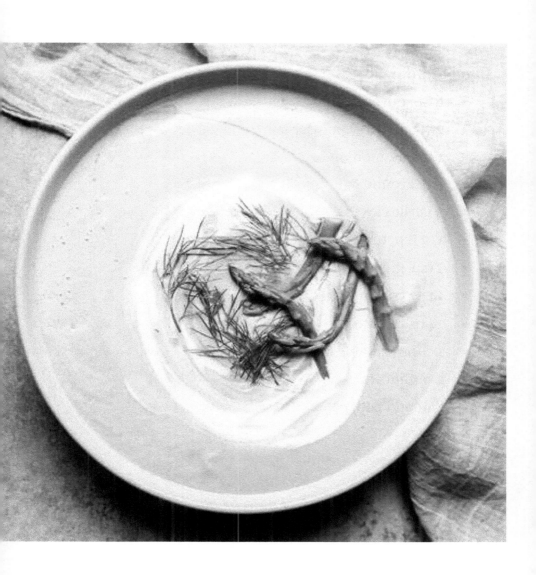

Coconut Curry Cauliflower Soup

Preparation Time: 15 minutes

Cooking Time: 30 minutes

Servings: 4

Ingredients:

- tbsp. olive oil
- 2-3 tsp. curry powder
- 1 medium onion
- tsp. ground cumin
- 3 garlic cloves
- 1/2 tsp. turmeric powder
- 1 tsp. ginger
- 14 oz coconut milk
- 14 oz tomatoes
- 1 cup vegetable broth
- 1 cauliflower
- Salt and pepper

Directions:

1. Take a pot, adds olive oil and onion, and set it on a medium flame for sautéing.
2. After 3 minutes, add garlic, ginger, curry powder, cumin, and turmeric powder and sauté for more than 5 minutes.

3. Now add coconut milk, tomatoes, vegetable broth, and cauliflower and mix it well.

4. Let the mixture heat and bring to boil.

5. Now on low flame, cook it for at least 20 minutes until cauliflower turns soft, blend the mixture well through a blender and heat the soup for more than 5 minutes, and add salt and pepper as per taste, serve the hot seasonal soup.

Nutrition:

Calories: 281 Fat: 8.1g Fiber: 3.8g Carbohydrates: 3.2 g Protein: 4.8g

Gazpacho Soup

Preparation Time: 25 minutes

Cooking Time: 0 minutes

Servings: 3

Ingredients:

- 1 large cucumber (to be sliced into chunks)
- 4 big ripe tomatoes (coarsely chopped)
- 1/2 bell pepper (any color)
- 2 cloves of garlic (minced)
- 1 celery rib (chopped)
- 1 tablespoon of lemon juice
- 1/4 tablespoon of celery pepper
- 1 tablespoon of fresh basil (chopped)
- 1 tablespoon of fresh parsley (chopped) Dash black pepper
- 1/2 tablespoon salt
- 3 tablespoons of red wine (vinegar/balsamic vinegar)
- 1/2 sweet onions (quartered)

Directions:

1. To make the gazpacho, place the cucumber chunks, chopped tomatoes, bell pepper, garlic, celery, lemon juice, and onion in the food processor or blender.
2. You may choose to blend or process in batches if needed

3. Add the vinegar (red/balsamic), salt, pepper to the blender or food processor and blend or process together until it is smooth or nearly smooth (the texture depends on you)

4. The next step is to pour soup into a serving bowl and stir in the fresh chopped parsley and basil

5. Cover the serving bowl with plastic wrap or foil or cover it with a plastic wrap and put the bowl inside the refrigerator for about 30 minutes or until when you are set to serve the gazpacho soup.

6. You can decide to add some extra fresh herbs to the soup for presentation as well as some avocado slices or crusty croutons

7. Serve gazpacho soup with a green salad, some artisanal or homemade bread as a substitute, balsamic vinegar, and olive oil for dipping for a light, but complete meal.

8. Serve and enjoy!

Nutrition:

Calories: 131 Fat: 9.4g Fiber: 16.8g Carbohydrates: 2.4 g Protein: 4.1g

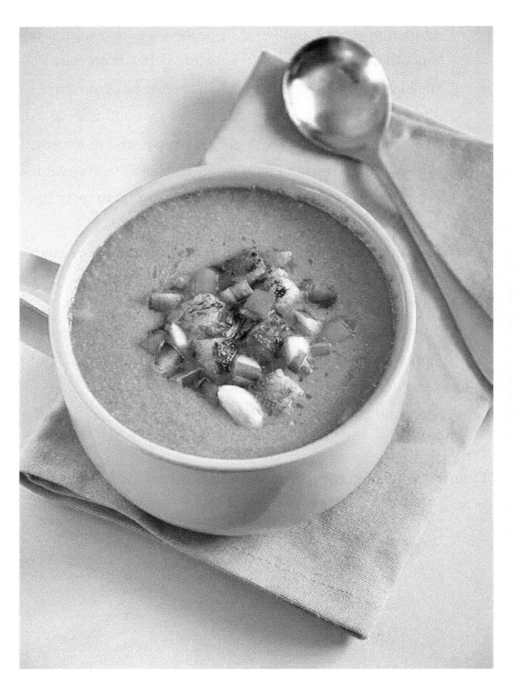

MAIN

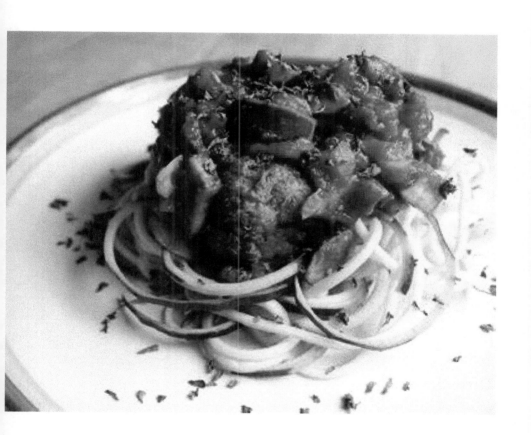

Zoodle Bolognese

Servings: 4

Cooking Time: 45 minutes

Ingredients

- 3 oz olive oil
- 1 white onion, chopped
- 1 garlic clove, minced
- 3 oz carrots, chopped
- 3 cups crumbled tofu
- 2 tbsp tomato paste
- 1 ½ cups crushed tomatoes
- Salt and black pepper to taste
- 1 tbsp dried basil
- 1 tbsp Worcestershire sauce
- 2 lbs zucchini, spiralized
- 2 tbsp vegan butter

Directions:

1. Heat olive oil in a saucepan and sauté onion, garlic, and carrots for 3 minutes.

2. Pour in tofu, tomato paste, tomatoes, salt, pepper, basil, some water, and Worcestershire sauce. Stir and cook for minutes.

3. Melt vegan butter in a skillet and toss in zoodles quickly, about 1 minute.

4. Season with salt and pepper.

5. Serve zoodles topped with the sauce.

Nutrition Info (Per Serving): Cal 425; Net Carbs 6g; Fat 33g; Protein 20g

Meatless Florentine Pizza

Servings: 2

Cooking Time: 35 minutes

Ingredients

- 1 cup shredded provolone cheese
- 1 (7 oz) can sliced mushrooms, drained
- 10 eggs
- 1 tsp Italian seasoning
- 2/3 cup tomato sauce
- 2 cups chopped kale, wilted
- ½ cup grated mozzarella
- 4 eggs

Directions:

1. Preheat oven to 400° F and line a pizza-baking pan with parchment paper.

2. Whisk 6 eggs with provolone cheese and Italian seasoning.

3. Spread the mixture on a pizza-baking pan, bake for minutes; let cool for 2 minutes. Increase the oven's temperature to 450° F.

4. Spread tomato sauce on the crust, top with kale, mozzarella cheese, and mushrooms.

5. Bake for 8 minutes. Crack remaining eggs on top and continue baking until the eggs are set, 3 minutes.

Nutrition Info (Per Serving): Cal 646; Net Carbs 4.9g; Fat 39g; Protein 36g

Parmesan Eggplant Casserole

Servings: 3

Preparation Time: 10 minutes

Cooking Time: 45 minutes

Ingredients:

- Eggplants -peeled, sliced: 1 ½ lb.
- Parmesan cheese -shredded: 1 cup
- Mozzarella cheese -shredded: 2 cups
- Low-carb spaghetti sauce-no-added sugar: 1 ½ cup
- Dried oregano: as required
- Dried basil: as required

Directions:

1. Grease a casserole dish and layer half the eggplant over it.
2. Sprinkle ¾ cup Mozzarella cheese, ½ cup Parmesan cheese, and ¾ cup sauce along with the spices.
3. Repeat the layering and sprinkle spices.
4. Cover using an aluminum foil and bake for 40 minutes at 375 degrees Fahrenheit.
5. Uncover and sprinkle the ½ cup Mozzarella cheese that is left along with some spices.
6. Bake for an additional 5 minutes.

Nutrition Value:

422.1 Cal, 26.7 g total fat -15.7 g sat. fat, 88.3 mg chol., 982.4 mg sodium, 15.9 g carbs, 7.7 g fiber, 31.7 g protein.

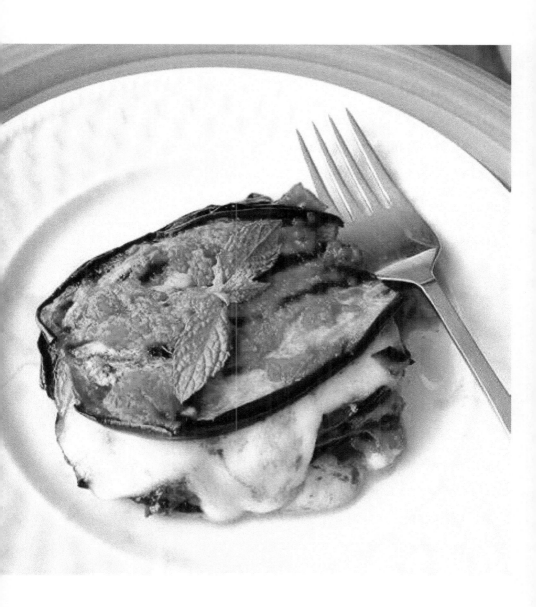

Noodle Bowl with Creamy Curry Sauce

Servings: 4

Preparation Time: 10 minutes

Cooking Time: 2 minutes

Ingredients:

- Cauliflower head -chopped roughly: ½
- Red bell pepper -diced: 1
- Fresh cilantro -chopped: handful
- Mixed greens - 2 handfuls

Sauce:

- Tahini: ¼ cup
- Apple cider vinegar: 2 tablespoon
- Water: ¼ cup
- Avocado oil: 2 tablespoon
- Curry powder: 2 teaspoon
- Ground coriander: 1 ½ teaspoon
- Ground turmeric: 1 teaspoon
- Ground cumin: 1 teaspoon
- Sea salt: 1 teaspoon
- Ground black pepper: ½ teaspoon
- Ground ginger: ¼ teaspoon

Directions:

1. Place all the sauce ingredients in a blender and blend until smooth.

2. For the noodles, place the noodle sheets in a bowl and pour warm water over it. Strain after 5 minutes and place in a large bowl.

3. Toss together all the ingredients and top with the sauce.

Nutrition Value:

192 Cal, 15.4 g total fat -2.1 g sat. fat, 7.3 g net. carbs, 10.4 g fiber, 4.3 g protein.

MEAT

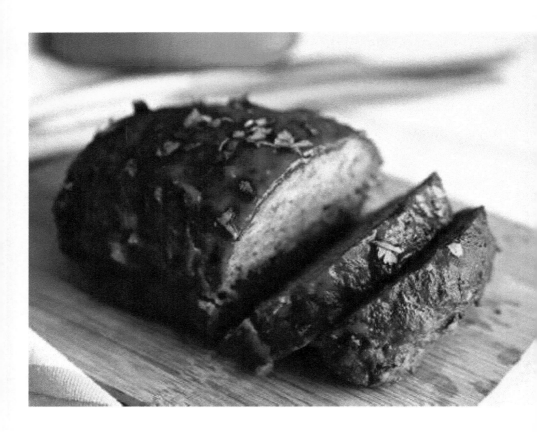

Cheddar Zucchini & Beef Mugs

Servings: 2

Cooking Time: 10 minutes

Ingredients

- 4 oz roast beef deli slices, torn apart
- 3 tbsp sour cream
- 1 small zucchini, chopped
- 2 tbsp chopped green chilies
- 3 oz shredded cheddar cheese

Directions:

1. Divide the beef slices at the bottom of 2 wide mugs and spread tbsp of sour cream.

2. Top with 2 zucchini slices, season with salt and pepper, add green chilies, top with the remaining sour cream and then cheddar cheese. Place the mugs in the microwave for 1-2 minutes until the cheese melts. Remove the mugs, let cool for 1 minute, and serve.

Nutrition Info (Per Serving): Cal 188; Net Carbs 3.7g; Fat 9g; Protein 18g

Grilled Beef Short Loin

Servings: 3

Cooking Time: 30 minutes

Ingredients

- 1 ½ pound beef short loin
- 2 thyme sprigs, chopped
- 1 rosemary sprig, chopped
- 1 teaspoon garlic powder
- Sea salt and ground black pepper, to taste

Directions:

1. Place all of the above ingredients in a re-sealable zipper bag. Shake until the short beef loin is well coated on all sides.

2. Cook on a preheated grill for 15 minutes, flipping once or twice during the cooking time.

3. Let it stand for 5 minutes before slicing and serving. Bon appétit!

Nutrition Info (Per Serving): 313 Calories; 11.6g Fat; 0.1g Carbs; 52g Protein; 0.1g Fiber

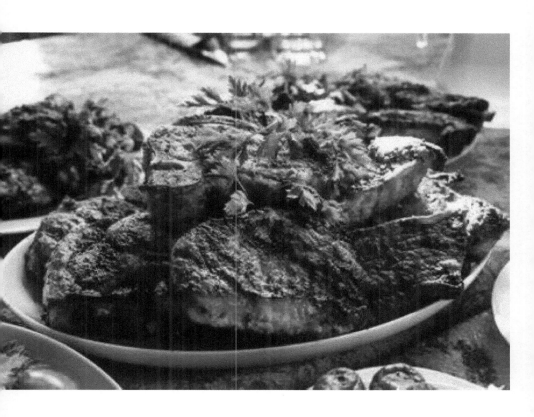

Herby Beef & Veggie Stew

Servings: 4

Cooking Time: 30 minutes

Ingredients

- 1 pound ground beef
- 2 tbsp olive oil
- 1 onion, chopped
- 2 garlic cloves, minced
- 14 ounces canned diced tomatoes
- 1 tbsp dried rosemary
- 1 tbsp dried sage
- 1 tbsp dried oregano
- 1 tbsp dried basil
- 1 tbsp dried marjoram
- Salt and black pepper, to taste
- 2 carrots, sliced
- 2 celery stalks, chopped
- 1 cup vegetable broth

Directions:

1. Set a pan over medium heat, add olive oil, onion, celery, garlic, and sauté for 5 minutes.

2. Place in the beef, and cook for 6 minutes. Stir in the tomatoes, carrots, broth, black pepper, oregano,

marjoram, basil, rosemary, salt, and sage, and simmer for minutes. Serve and enjoy!

Nutrition Info (Per Serving): Kcal 253, Fat 13g, Net Carbs 5.2g, Protein 30g

Sausage with Zucchini Noodles

Servings: 2

Cooking Time: 12 minutes

Ingredients

- 1 large zucchini, spiralized into noodles
- 3 oz sausage
- ½ tsp garlic powder
- 4 oz marinara sauce
- 2 tsp grated parmesan cheese
- Seasoning:
- 1/3 tsp salt
- 1/8 tsp dried basil
- ¼ tsp Italian seasoning
- 1 tbsp avocado oil

Directions:

1. Take a skillet pan, place it over medium heat and when hot, add sausage, crumble it and cook for 5 minutes until nicely browned.

2. When done, transfer sausage to a bowl, drain the grease, add oil and when hot, add zucchini noodles, sprinkle with garlic, toss until mixed and cook for 3 minutes until zucchini begins to tender.

3. Add marinara sauce, return sausage into the pan, toss until mixed, add salt, basil and Italian seasoning, stir until mixed and cook for 2 to 3 minutes until hot. When done, distribute marinara noodles between two plates, sprinkle with cheese and then serve.

Nutrition Info: 320 Calories; 27.6 g Fats; 8.6 g Protein; 5.2 g Net Carb; 2.7 g Fiber

Ultimate Zucchini Lasagna

Servings: 7

Cooking Time: 45 minutes

Ingredients

- 2 tablespoons olive oil
- 2 ½ pounds ground chuck
- 1 shallot, chopped
- Sea salt and ground black pepper, to taste
- 1 teaspoon cayenne pepper
- 1 tablespoon steak seasoning blend
- 1 large-sized zucchini, sliced
- 7 eggs
- 7 ounces cream cheese
- 1 cup Asiago cheese, shredded

Directions:

1. Heat the olive oil in a frying pan over a moderate flame; once hot, brown the ground chuck for 4 to 5 minutes.

2. Add in the shallot and continue to sauté for 3 minutes more or until tender and translucent. Season with salt, black pepper, cayenne pepper, and steak seasoning blend.

3. Pat dry the zucchini slices to get rid of the excess moisture.

4. Spoon 1/3 of the mixture into the bottom of a lightly greased casserole dish. Top with the layer of zucchini slices. Repeat until you run out of zucchini and beef mixture.

5. In a mixing bowl, whisk the eggs with the sour cream; spread the mixture on top. Top with the Asiago cheese.

6. Cover the casserole dish with aluminum foil. Bake in the preheated oven at 3 degrees F for 20 minutes.

7. Remove the aluminum foil and bake for a further 15 minutes until the top is golden. Bon appétit!

Nutrition Info (Per Serving): 467 Calories; 31.8g Fat; 3.3g Carbs; 42g Protein; 0.4g Fiber

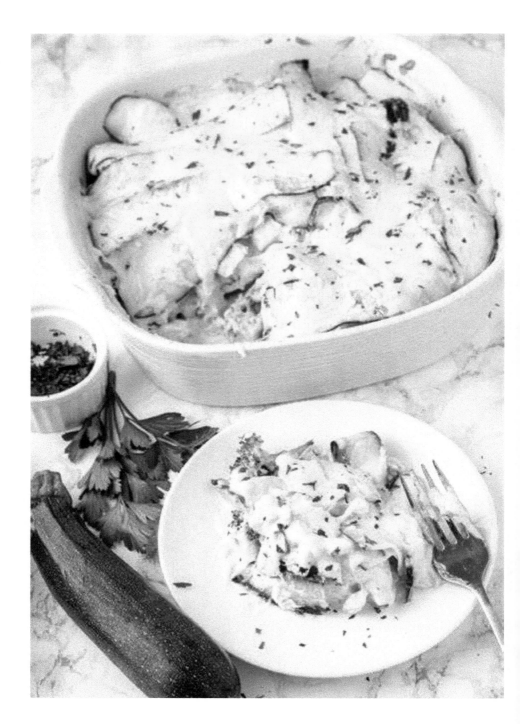

Tarragon Beef Meatloaf

Servings: 4

Cooking Time: 70 minutes

Ingredients

- 2 lb ground beef
- 3 tbsp flaxseed meal
- 2 large eggs
- 2 tbsp olive oil
- 1 lemon, zested
- ¼ cup chopped tarragon
- ¼ cup chopped oregano
- 4 garlic cloves, minced

Directions:

1. Preheat the oven to 400° F and grease a loaf pan with cooking spray. In a bowl, combine beef, salt, pepper, and flaxseed meal; set aside.

2. In another bowl, whisk the eggs with olive oil, lemon zest, tarragon, oregano, and garlic. Pour the mixture onto the beef mix and evenly combine.

3. Spoon the meat mixture into the pan and press to fit in. Bake in the oven for an hour. Remove the pan, tilt to drain the meat's liquid, and let cool for 5 minutes.

4. Slice, garnish with some lemon slices and serve with curried cauli rice.

Nutrition Info (Per Serving): Cal 631; Net Carbs 2.8g; Fat 38g; Protein 64g

Sausage with Tomatoes and Cheese

Servings: 4

Cooking Time: 30 minutes

Ingredients

- 2 ounces coconut oil, melted
- 2 pounds Italian pork sausage, chopped
- 1 onion, sliced
- 4 sun-dried tomatoes, thinly sliced
- Salt and black pepper to the taste
- ½ pound gouda cheese, grated
- 3 yellow bell peppers, chopped
- 3 orange bell peppers, chopped
- A pinch of red pepper flakes
- A handful parsley, thinly sliced

Directions:

1. Heat up a pan with the oil over medium-high heat, add sausage slices, stir, cook for 3 minutes on each side, transfer to a plate and leave aside for now.
2. Heat up the pan again over medium heat, add onion, yellow and orange bell peppers and tomatoes, stir and cook for 5 minutes.
3. Add pepper flakes, salt and pepper, stir well, cook for 1 minute and take off the heat.

4. Arrange sausage slices into a baking dish, add bell peppers mix on top, add parsley and gouda as well, introduce in the oven at 350 degrees F and bake for 15 minutes.

5. Divide between plates and serve hot.

6. Enjoy!

Nutrition Info: calories 200, fat 5, fiber 3, carbs 6, protein 14

Tuscan Pork Tenderloin with Cauli Rice

Servings: 4

Cooking Time: 30 minutes

Ingredients

- 1 cup loosely packed fresh baby spinach
- 2 tbsp olive oil
- 1 ½ lb pork tenderloin, cubed
- Salt and black pepper to taste
- ½ tsp cumin powder
- 2 cups cauliflower rice
- ½ cup of water
- 1 cup grape tomatoes, halved
- 3/4 cup crumbled feta cheese

Directions:

1. In a skillet, heat olive oil, season the pork with salt, pepper, and cumin, and sear on both sides for 5 minutes until brown. Stir in cauli rice and pour in water.

2. Cook for 5 minutes or until cauliflower softens. Mix in spinach to wilt, minute, and add the tomatoes. Spoon the dish into bowls, sprinkle with feta cheese, and serve with hot sauce.

Nutrition Info (Per Serving): Cal 377; Net Carbs 1.9g; Fat 17g; Protein 43g

Chunky Hamburger Soup

Servings: 7

Cooking Time: 1 Hour

Ingredients

- 2 tablespoons sesame oil
- 2 ½ pounds ground chuck
- 1 yellow onion, chopped
- 1/2 teaspoon fresh or dried basil
- 1 teaspoon fresh coriander, minced
- 1 teaspoon garlic powder
- Kosher salt and black pepper, to season
- 1 stalk celery, chopped
- 2 ripe tomatoes, pureed
- 1 bay laurel
- 8 cups of water
- 3 bouillon cubes

Directions:

1. Heat the sesame oil in a soup pot over a medium-high flame. Once hot, brown the ground chuck for 4 to 5 minutes, crumbling with a fork.

2. Add in the onion and continue to sauté for about 4 minutes. Stir in the remaining ingredients; gently stir to combine.

3. Turn the heat to medium-low and let it simmer, partially covered, for 50 minutes or until cooked through.

4. Taste, adjust the seasonings, and serve in individual bowls. Bon appétit!

Nutrition Info (Per Serving): 301 Calories; 17.7g Fat; 3.3g Carbs; 32.5g Protein; 0.8g Fiber

POULTRY

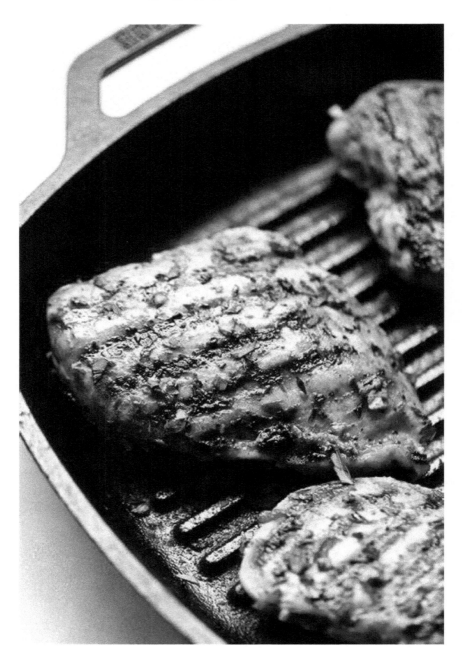

Parsnip & Bacon Chicken Bake

Servings: 4

Cooking Time: 50 minutes

Ingredients

- 6 bacon slices, chopped
- 2 tbsp butter
- ½ lb parsnips, diced
- 2 tbsp olive oil
- 1 lb ground chicken
- 2 tbsp butter
- 1 cup heavy cream
- 2 oz cream cheese, softened
- 1 ¼ cups grated Pepper Jack
- ¼ cup chopped scallions

Directions:

1. Preheat oven to 300° F. Put the bacon in a pot and fry until brown and crispy, 7 minutes; set aside. Melt butter in a skillet and sauté parsnips until softened and lightly browned. Transfer to a greased baking sheet. Heat olive oil in the same pan and cook the chicken until no longer pink, 8 minutes. Spoon onto a plate and set aside too.

2. Add heavy cream, cream cheese, two-thirds of the Pepper Jack cheese, salt, and pepper to the pot. Melt the

63

ingredients over medium heat, frequently stirring, 7 minutes. Spread the parsnips on the baking dish, top with chicken, pour the heavy cream mixture over, and scatter bacon and scallions. Sprinkle the remaining cheese on top and bake until the cheese melts and is golden, 30 minutes.

Nutrition Info (Per Serving): Cal 757; Net Carbs 5.5g; Fat 66g; Protein 29g

Parmesan Chicken and Kale Sauté

Servings: 2

Cooking Time: 10 minutes

Ingredients

- 2 chicken thighs, boneless, cut into strips
- ½ bunch of kale
- 1 tsp garlic powder
- 1 tbsp avocado oil
- 4 tbsp grated parmesan cheese

Seasoning:

- 1/3 tsp salt
- 1/4 tsp ground black pepper
- 1/3 tsp red pepper flakes

Directions:

1. Take a medium skillet pan, place it over medium heat, add oil and when hot, add chicken in it, season with salt and black pepper and cook for 5 minutes until thoroughly cooked.

2. Transfer chicken to a plate, add kale into the pan, sprinkle with garlic and red pepper flakes and cook for 3 to 4 minutes until kale is just tender.

3. Return chicken into the pan, stir until mixed, sprinkle with parmesan cheese, stir until combined, and remove the pan from heat. Serve.

Nutrition Info: 303.3 Calories; 15.7 g Fats; 31.6 g Protein; 5 g Net Carb; 3.9 g Fiber

Cranberry Glazed Chicken with Onions

Servings: 6

Cooking Time: 50 minutes

Ingredients

- 4 green onions, chopped diagonally
- 4 tbsp unsweetened cranberry puree
- 2 lb chicken wings
- 2 tbsp olive oil
- Chili sauce to taste
- Juice from 1 lime

Directions:

1. Preheat the oven (broiler side) to 400 F. Then, in a bowl, mix the cranberry puree, olive oil, salt, sweet chili sauce, and lime juice. After, add in the wings and toss to coat. Place the chicken under the broiler, and cook for 45 minutes, turning once halfway. Remove the chicken after and serve warm with a cranberry puree and cheese dipping sauce.

2. Top with green onions to serve.

Nutrition Info (Per Serving): Cal 152, Net Carbs 1.6g, Fat 8.5g, Protein 17g

Oregano & Chili Flattened Chicken
Servings: 6

Cooking Time: 5 minutes

Ingredients

- 6 chicken breasts
- 4 cloves garlic, minced
- ½ cup oregano leaves, chopped
- ½ cup lemon juice
- 2/3 cup olive oil
- ¼ cup erythritol
- Salt and black pepper to taste
- 3 small chilies, minced

Directions:

1. Preheat a grill to 350° F.

2. In a bowl, mix the garlic, oregano, lemon juice, olive oil, chilies and erythritol. Set aside.

3. While the spices incorporate in flavor, cover the chicken with plastic wraps, and use the rolling pin to pound to ½ - inch thickness. Remove the wrap, and brush the mixture on the chicken on both sides.

4. Place on the grill, cover the lid and cook for 15 minutes. Baste the chicken with more of the spice mixture, and continue cooking for 15 more minutes.

Nutrition Info (Per Serving): Kcal 265, Fat 9g, Net Carbs 3g, Protein 26g

FISH

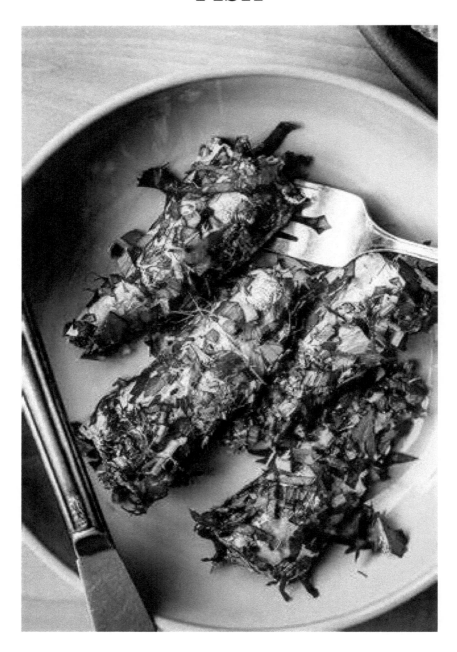

Incredible Salmon Dish

Servings: 4

Cooking Time: 15 minutes

Ingredients

- 3 cups of ice water
- 2 teaspoons sriracha sauce
- 4 teaspoons stevia
- 3 scallions, chopped
- Salt and black pepper to the taste
- 2 teaspoons flaxseed oil
- 4 teaspoons apple cider vinegar
- 3 teaspoons avocado oil
- 4 medium salmon fillets
- 4 cups baby arugula
- 2 cups cabbage, finely chopped
- 1 and ½ teaspoon Jamaican jerk seasoning
- ¼ cup pepitas, toasted
- 2 cups watermelon radish, julienned

Directions:

1. Put ice water in a bowl, add scallions and leave aside.
2. In another bowl, mix sriracha sauce with stevia and stir well.

3. Transfer 2 teaspoons of this mix to a bowl and mix with half of the avocado oil, flaxseed oil, vinegar, salt and pepper and whisk well.

4. Sprinkle jerk seasoning over salmon, rub with sriracha and stevia mix and season with salt and pepper.

5. Heat up a pan with the other half of the avocado oil over medium-high heat, add salmon, flesh side down, cook for 4 minutes, flip and cook for 4 minutes more and divide between plates.

6. In a bowl, mix radishes with cabbage and arugula.

7. Add salt, pepper, sriracha and vinegar mix and toss well.

8. Add this next to salmon fillets, drizzle the remaining sriracha and stevia sauce all over and top with pepitas and drained scallions.

9. Enjoy!

Nutrition Info: calories 160, fat 6, fiber 1, carbs 1, protein 12

Fish Curry Masala

Servings: 6

Cooking Time: 25 minutes

Ingredients

- 2 tablespoons sesame oil
- 1 shallot, chopped
- 2 bell peppers, deveined and sliced
- 1 teaspoon coriander, ground
- 1 teaspoon cumin, ground
- 4 tablespoons red curry paste
- 1 teaspoon ginger-garlic paste
- 1 ½ pound white fish fillets, skinless, boneless
- 1/2 cup tomato sauce
- 1/2 cup haddi ka shorba Indian bone broth
- 1 cup coconut milk
- 1/2 teaspoon red chili powder
- Salt and ground black pepper, to taste

Directions:

1. Heat the sesame oil in a saucepan over moderate heat; then, sauté the shallot and peppers until they have softened or about 4 minutes.

2. Now, stir in the coriander, cumin, red curry paste, and ginger-garlic paste; continue to sauté an additional 4 minutes, stirring frequently.

3. After that, fold in the fish and tomato sauce; pour in the haddi ka shorba and coconut milk. Season with red chili powder, salt, and black pepper.

4. Turn the heat to simmer and let it cook for 5 minutes longer or until everything is cooked through. Enjoy!

Nutrition Info (Per Serving): 349 Calories; 24.9g Fat; 6.2g Carbs; 22.7g Protein; 2.5g Fiber

Indian Chepala Vepudu

Servings: 3

Cooking Time: 15 minutes

Ingredients

- 3 carp fillets
- 1 teaspoon chili powder
- 1 teaspoon cumin powder
- 1 teaspoon turmeric powder
- 1 coriander powder
- 1/2 teaspoon garam masala
- 1/2 teaspoon flaky salt
- 1/4 teaspoon cayenne pepper
- 3 tablespoons full-fat coconut milk
- 1 egg
- 2 tablespoons olive oil
- 6 curry leaves, for garnish

Directions:

1. Pat, the fish, fillets with kitchen towels and add them to a large resealable bag. Add the spices to the bag and shake to coat on all sides.

2. In a shallow dish, whisk the coconut milk and egg until frothy and well combined. Dip the fillets into the egg mixture.

3. Then, heat the oil in a large frying pan. Fry the fish fillets on both sides until they are cooked through and the coating becomes crispy.

4. Serve with curry leaves and enjoy!

Nutrition Info (Per Serving): 443 Calories; 28.3g Fat; 2.6g Carbs; 42.5g Protein; 1g Fiber

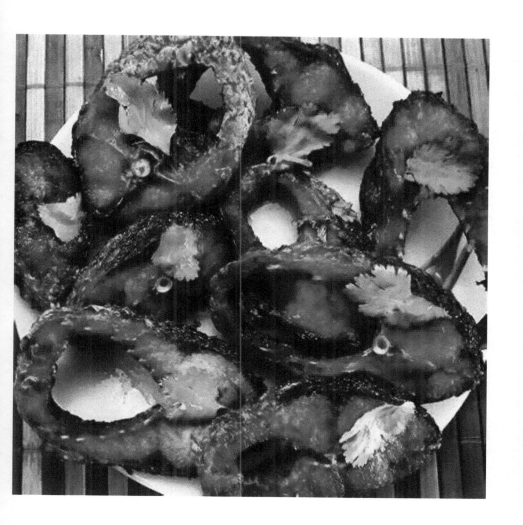

Shrimp in Curry Sauce

Servings: 2

Cooking Time: 15 minutes

Ingredients

- ½ ounce grated Parmesan cheese
- 1 egg, beaten
- ¼ tsp curry powder
- 2 tsp almond flour
- 12 shrimp, shelled
- 3 tbsp coconut oil

Sauce

- 2 tbsp curry leaves
- 2 tbsp butter
- ½ onion, diced
- ½ cup heavy cream
- ½ ounce cheddar cheese, shredded

Directions:

1. Combine all dry ingredients for the batter. Melt the coconut oil in a skillet over medium heat. Dip the shrimp in the egg first, and then coat with the dry mixture. Fry until golden and crispy.

2. In another skillet, melt butter. Add onion and cook for 3 minutes. Add curry leaves and cook for 30 seconds. Stir in

heavy cream and cheddar and cook until thickened. Add shrimp and coat well. Serve.

Nutrition Info (Per Serving): Kcal 560, Fat: 41g, Net Carbs: 4.3g, Protein: 24.4g

Herbed Sardines

Servings: 4

Cooking Time: 8 minutes

Ingredients

- 12 2-ounces fresh sardines, cleaned and scaled
- Salt and ground black pepper, as required
- 2 tablespoons olive oil
- ½ cup green olives, pitted and chopped
- 2 cups fresh parsley leaves, chopped
- 1 tablespoon fresh oregano, chopped
- 2 tablespoons capers, drained
- 2 garlic cloves, thinly sliced
- 2 Serrano peppers, seeded and minced
- 1 teaspoon lemon zest, grated finely

Directions:

1. Preheat the oven to 400 degrees F.
2. Lightly, season the sardines with salt and black pepper.
3. Heat the olive oil in a large ovenproof skillet and cook the sardines for about minutes.
4. Flip the sardines and stir in the remaining ingredients.
5. Immediately transfer the skillet into the oven and bake for about minutes or until the fish's desired doneness.

6. Remove from oven and transfer the fish mixture onto serving plates.

7. Serve hot.

Nutrition Info (Per Serving): Calories: 452; Net Carbs: 2.4g; Carbohydrate: 4.7g; Fiber: 2.3g; Protein: 43.3g; Fat: 28.7g; Sugar: 0.5g; Sodium: 1180mg

Traditional New Orleans Gumbo

Servings: 6

Cooking Time: 30 minutes

Ingredients

- 3 teaspoons butter, at room temperature
- 1 pound andouille sausage, sliced
- 1 red onion, chopped
- 2 cloves garlic, minced
- 1 celery stalk, chopped
- 1 red chili pepper, chopped
- 2 pounds halibut, cut into bite-sized chunks
- 2 tomatoes, pureed
- 4 cups of water
- 3 cubes beef bouillon
- 1/2 teaspoon Cajun seasoning blend
- Flaky salt and ground black pepper, to taste
- 1 pound lump crabmeat
- 1 teaspoon cayenne pepper
- 1 tbsp fresh cilantro

Directions:

1. Melt a teaspoon of the butter in a heavy-bottomed pot over a moderate flame. Now, brown the sausage for 2 to 3 minutes; reserve.

2. Melt the remaining teaspoons of butter and add in the red onion, garlic, celery, and chili pepper; let it cook for 1 ½ minute more.

3. Now, stir in the halibut, tomatoes, water, cubes of beef bouillon and bring to a boil. Reduce the heat and let it simmer, partially covered, for 1minutes.

4. Then, stir in the Cajun seasoning blend, salt, ground black pepper, crabmeat, and cayenne pepper; return the sausage to the pot.

5. Stir to combine well and let it cook for 6 minutes more. Ladle into individual bowls and serve garnished with fresh cilantro. Enjoy!

Nutrition Info (Per Serving): 441 Calories; 27.5g Fat; 5.9g Carbs; 39.8g Protein; 1.2g Fiber

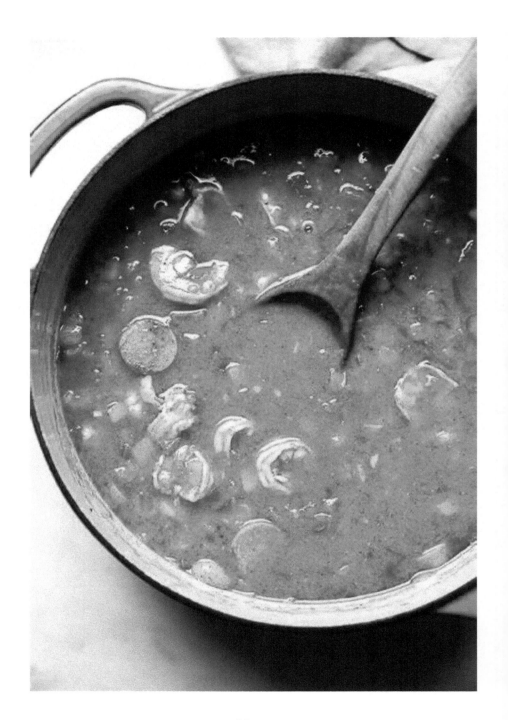

Salmon with Roasted Veggies

Servings: 2

Cooking Time: 15 minutes

Ingredients

- 2 fillets of salmon4 oz asparagus spears cut
- 2 oz sliced mushrooms
- 2 oz grape tomatoes
- 2 oz basil pesto

Seasoning:

- 2/3 tsp salt
- ½ tsp ground black pepper
- 1 tbsp mayonnaise
- 1.5 oz grated mozzarella cheese
- 2 tbsp avocado oil

Directions:

1. Turn on the oven, then set it to 425 degrees F and let it preheat. Take a medium baking sheet lined with parchment paper, place salmon fillets on it and then season with 3 tsp salt and ¼ tsp ground black pepper.
2. Take a small bowl, mix together mayonnaise and pesto in it until combined, spread this mixture over seasoned salmon and then top evenly with cheese.

3. Take a medium bowl, place all the vegetables in it, season with remaining salt and black pepper, drizzle with oil and toss until coated.

4. Spread vegetables around prepared fillets and then bake for 12 to 15 minutes until fillets have thoroughly cooked. Serve.

Nutrition Info: 571 Calories; 45.4 g Fats; 34.1 g Protein; 3.5 g Net Carb; 2.2 g Fiber

VEGETABLES

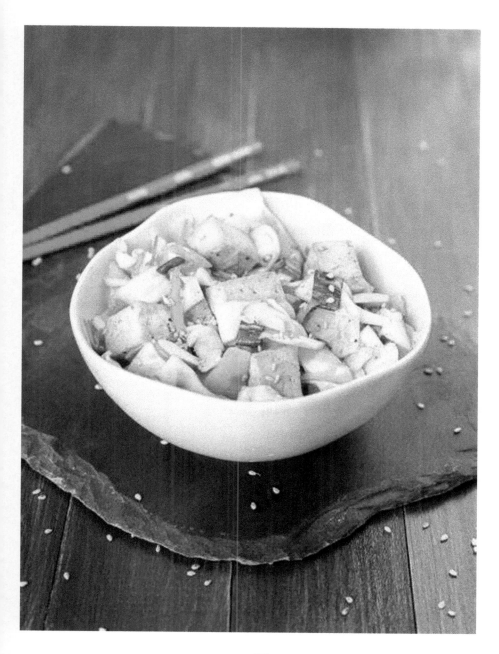

Tofu Salad

Preparation Time: 15 minutes

Cooking Time: 30 minutes

Servings: 4

Ingredients:

- 15oz. extra firm drained tofu
- 1 tablespoon coconut aminos
- 1 tablespoon coconut oil
- 2 teaspoons minced garlic
- 1 tablespoon of filtered water
- ½ lemon juice

For the salad:

- 9oz. fresh Bok Choy
- 3 tablespoons extra-virgin coconut oil
- 2 tablespoons coconut aminos
- 2 tablespoons chopped parsley
- 1 tablespoon almond butter
- 1 tablespoon ground chili sambal

Directions:

1. Make the tofu; cut tofu into squares and place in a bowl.
2. In a small bowl, whisk coconut aminos, coconut oil, garlic, water, and lemon juice. Pour mixture over tofu and toss gently to combine. Cover and refrigerate for 1 hour.

3. Heat oven to 350F and line a baking sheet with parchment paper. Arrange the tofu on a baking sheet and bake for 30 minutes.

4. Make the Bok choy; in a bowl, combine all ingredients except Bok choy and lemon juice.

5. Just before tofu is baked, stir in lemon juice. Chop the Bok choy and stir into prepared dressing.

6. Remove tofu cubes from the oven and serve with Bok choy.

Brilliant Cheesy Broccoli

Preparation Time: 25 minutes

Servings: 2

Ingredients:

For Broccoli:

- 2 cups broccoli florets
- 1 tbsp. olive oil
- 2 tsp garlic powder
- ½ tbsp. smoked paprika
- Salt and freshly ground black pepper, to taste

For Cheese Sauce:

- tbsp. butter
- 2 tbs. almond flour
- ½ cups unsweetened almond milk
- 1 cup shredded cheddar cheese
- 1 tsp garlic powder
- Salt, to taste

Directions:

1. For the broccoli: in a bowl, add all ingredients and toss to coat well.
2. In the bottom of the Instant Pot, arrange a steamer basket and pour 1 cup of water.

3. Place the broccoli into the steamer basket.

4. Secure the lid and place the pressure valve in the "Seal" position.

5. Select "Manual" and cook under "Low Pressure" for about 10 minutes.

6. Select the "Cancel" and carefully do a "Natural" release.

7. Meanwhile, for cheese sauce: In a medium pan, melt butter over medium-high heat.

8. Add flour, beating continuously.

9. Slowly add almond milk, beating continuously.

10. Cook for about 2-3 minutes or until thickened, stirring continuously.

11. Add cheese, garlic powder, and salt and stir until smooth.

12. Remove the lid of Instant Pot and transfer broccoli onto serving plates.

13. To wit cheese sauce and serve.

Nutrition Values:

Calories 536, Total Fat 47.9g, Net Carbs 5g, Protein 19.3g, Fiber 4.3g

Better-Than-Real Mash

Preparation Time: 18 minutes

Servings: 8

Ingredients:

- ½ cup homemade chicken broth
- 1 chopped head cauliflower
- 2 tbsp. plain Greek yogurt
- Salt and ground black pepper, to taste
- 2 tsp melted butter
- 2 tbsp. chopped chives

Directions:

1. In the bottom of the Instant Pot, arrange a steamer basket and pour the broth.
2. Place the cauliflower into the steamer basket.
3. Secure the lid and place the pressure valve in the "Seal" position.
4. Select "Manual" and cook under "High Pressure" for about 3 minutes.
5. Select the "Cancel" and carefully do a "Quick" release.
6. Remove the lid and transfer the cauliflower into a food processor.
7. Add yogurt, salt, and black pepper, and pulse until smooth.
8. Transfer the mashed cauliflower to a serving bowl.

9. Drizzle with melted ghee and serve with the garnishing of chives.

Nutrition Values:

Calories 40, Total Fat 1.2g, Net Carbs 0.75g, Protein 2.7g, Fiber 2.7g

Spicy Cauliflower

Preparation Time: 22 minutes

Servings: 4

Ingredients:

- 2 roughly chopped tomatoes
- ½ chopped small onion
- 1 green chile
- 1 tsp olive oil
- 1 tsp ground cumin
- ½ tsp ground turmeric
- ½ tsp paprika
- Salt and freshly ground black pepper, to taste
- 1 cut into small florets large head cauliflower
- ½ cup water
- 1 tbsp. chopped fresh cilantro

Directions:

1. In a food processor, add tomato, onion, and green chile and pulse until smooth.
2. Place the oil in the Instant Pot and select "Sauté." Then add the pureed onion mixture and cook for about 2-3 minutes.
3. Add spices and cook for about 1 minute.
4. Select the "Cancel" and stir in cauliflower and water.

5. Secure the lid and place the pressure valve in the "Seal" position.

6. Select "Manual" and cook under "Low Pressure" for about 2-3 minutes.

7. Select the "Cancel" and carefully do a quick release.

8. Remove the lid and serve.

Nutrition Values:

Calories 74, Total Fat 1.7, Net Carbs 3.37g, Protein 4.5g, Fiber 5.8g

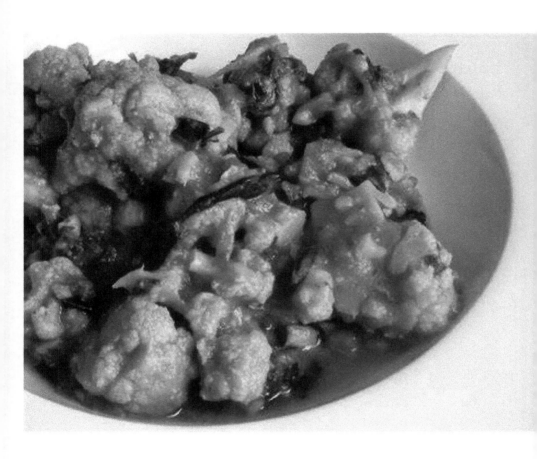

Creamy Radishes

Servings: 1

Cooking Time: 25 minutes

Ingredients

- 7 ounces radishes, cut in halves
- 2 tablespoons sour cream
- 2 bacon slices
- 1 tablespoon green onion, chopped
- 1 tablespoon cheddar cheese, grated
- Hot sauce to the taste
- Salt and black pepper to the taste

Directions:

1. Put radishes into a pot, add water to cover, bring to a boil over medium heat, cook them for minutes and drain.
2. Heat up a pan over medium-high heat, add bacon, cook until it's crispy, transfer to paper towels, drain grease, crumble and leave aside.
3. Return pan to medium heat, add radishes, stir and sauté them for 7 minutes. Add onion, salt, pepper, hot sauce and sour cream, stir and cook for 7 minutes more.
4. Transfer to a plate, top with crumbled bacon and cheddar cheese and serve. Enjoy!

Nutrition Info: calories 340, fat 23, fiber 3, carbs 6, protein 15

DESSERT

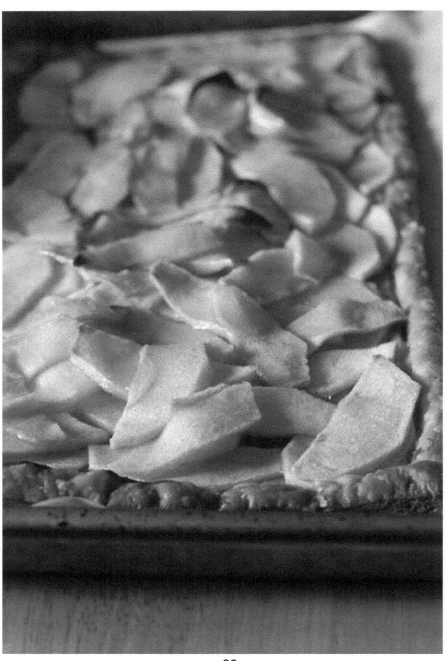

Chocolate Walnut Cookies

Preparation Time: 15 minutes

Cooking Time: 12 minutes

Servings: 6

Ingredients:

- 1/4 cup coconut oil
- 3 tbsp. sweetener
- 4 tbsp. unsalted butter
- 1 cup sugar-free chocolate chips
- 1 cup coconut flakes
- 1/2 cup pecans
- 1/2 cup walnuts
- 1 tsp. vanilla extract
- 4 egg yolks
- Sea salt

Directions:

1. Take a bowl and mix coconut oil, butter, sweetener, chocolate chips, vanilla extract, egg yolks, coconut, and walnuts, and stir well.
2. Use a scope to make a cookie and drop an even amount of dough on the baking pan.
3. Sprinkle salt as per taste and bake for 12 minutes on preheated oven at 350F until golden brown.

Nutrition:

Calories: 231 Fat: 7.4g Fiber: 3.1g Carbohydrates: 2.8 g Protein: 1.3g

Almond Shortbread Cookies

Preparation Time: 15 minutes

Cooking Time: 12 minutes

Servings: 6

Ingredients:

- 1/3 cup coconut flour
- 1/4 cup erythritol
- 2/3 cup almond flour
- 8 drops stevia
- 1/2 cup butter
- 1 tsp. almond or vanilla extract
- 1/4 tsp. baking powder

- For glaze:
- 1/4 cup coconut butter
- 8 drops stevia

Directions:

1. In a bowl, add coconut flour, almond flour, erythritol, baking powder, and add vanilla or almond extract, stevia, and melted butter and make a soft dough.
2. The dough must be divided into two and chill in the refrigerator for 10 minutes.

3. Roll the dough on a sheet and cut cookies with the help of a cookie cutter.

4. Place cookies into a baking pan and bake for 6 minutes in a preheated oven at 180C.

5. Now let the cookies completely cool and apply the glaze.

Nutrition:

Calories: 245 Fat: 9.4g Fiber: 3.1g Carbohydrates: 2.9 g Protein: 1.8g

Coconut Chia Pudding

Preparation Time: 10 minutes

Cooking Time: 0 minutes

Servings: 1

Ingredients:

- 1/4 cup chia seeds
- 1/4 cup coconut milk
- tbsp. unsweetened coconut
- 1 tsp. vanilla extract
- 2 tbsp. maple syrup

Directions:

1. Soak chia seeds in water for 2 to 3 minutes.
2. Take a bowl, add coconut milk, maple syrup, vanilla extract, and chia seeds and whisk them well.
3. Let it aside and mix again after 5 minutes.
4. Put it in an airtight bag and place it in the refrigerator for 1 hour. Serve and enjoy chilled coconut chia pudding.

Nutrition:

Calories: 165 Fat: 1.4g Fiber: 5.4g Carbohydrates: 1.2 g Protein: 3.1g

Granny Smith Apple Tart

Preparation Time: 15 minutes

Cooking Time: 25 minutes

Servings: 6

Ingredients:

- 6 tbsp. butter
- 2 cups almond flour
- 1 tsp. cinnamon
- 1/3 cup sweetener

Filling:

- 2 cups sliced Granny Smith
- 1/4 cup butter
- 1/4 cup sweetener
- 1/2 tsp. cinnamon
- 1/2 tsp. lemon juice

Topping:

- 1/4 tsp. cinnamon
- 2 tbsp. sweetener

Directions:

1. Preheat oven to 370°F and combine all crust ingredients in a bowl.

2. Press this mixture into the bottom of a greased pan. Bake for 5 minutes.

3. Meanwhile, combine the apples and lemon juice in a bowl and sit until the crust is ready.

4. Arrange them on top of the crust.

5. Combine remaining filling ingredients, and brush this mixture over the apples. Bake for about 30 minutes.

6. Press the apples down with a spatula, return to oven, and bake for 20 more minutes. Combine the cinnamon and sweetener in a bowl, and sprinkle over the tart.

Nutrition:

Calories: 276 Fat: 11g Fiber: 10.4g Carbohydrates: 2.1 g Protein: 3.1g

Dark Chocolate Fudge

Servings: 4

Cooking Time: 30 minutes

Ingredients

- 1 cup dark chocolate, melted
- 4 large eggs
- 1 cup swerve sugar
- ½ cup melted butter
- 1/3 cup coconut flour

Directions:

1. Preheat the oven to 350° F and line a rectangular baking tray with parchment paper. In a bowl, cream the eggs with swerving sugar until smooth.

2. Add in melted chocolate, butter, and whisk until evenly combined.

3. Carefully fold in the coconut flour to incorporate and pour the mixture into the baking tray.

4. Bake for 20 minutes or until a toothpick inserted comes out clean. Remove from the oven and allow cooling in the tray. Cut into squares and serve.

Nutrition Info (Per Serving): Cal 491; Net Carbs 2.8g, Fat 45g, Protein 13g

Avocado Truffles with Chocolate Coating

Servings: 6

Cooking Time: 5 minutes

Ingredients

- 1 ripe avocado, pitted
- ½ tsp vanilla extract
- ½ tsp lemon zest
- 5 oz dark chocolate
- 1 tbsp coconut oil
- 1 tbsp cocoa powder

Directions:

1. Scoop the pulp of the avocado into a bowl and mix with vanilla using an immersion blender. Stir in lemon zest and a pinch of salt.
2. Microwave chocolate and coconut oil for a minute.
3. Add to the avocado mixture and stir. Allow cooling to firm up a bit.
4. Form balls out of the mix.
5. Roll each ball in the cocoa powder and serve immediately.

Nutrition Info (Per Serving): Cal 70; Net Carbs 2g; Fat 6g; Protein 2g

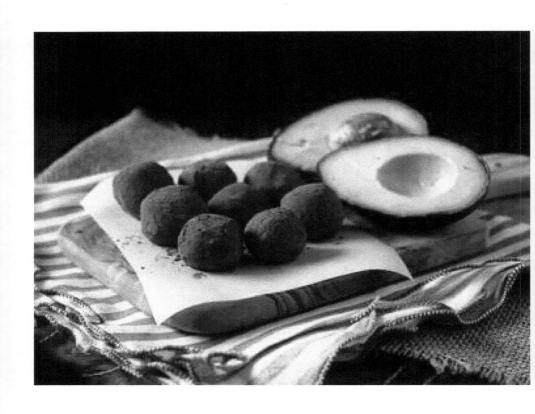

Lightning Source UK Ltd.
Milton Keynes UK
UKHW020635220621
385949UK00001B/42